GUT

GOODBYE

LEAKY GUT!

THE ULTIMATE SOLUTION FOR LEAKY GUT SYNDROME

DIGESTION - CANDIDA - IBS

Third Edition
SCOTT STERLING

© 2016

COPYRIGHT NOTICE

DISCLAIMER

Although the author and publisher have made every effort to ensure that the information in this book was correct at press time, the author and publisher do not assume and hereby disclaim any liability to any party for any loss, damage, or disruption caused by errors or omissions, whether such errors or omissions result from negligence, accident, or any other cause.

This book is not intended as a substitute for the medical advice of physicians. The reader should regularly consult a physician in matters relating to his/her health and particularly with respect to any symptoms that may require diagnosis or medical attention.

TABLE OF CONTENTS

INTRODUCTION

If you've ever gotten a random pain in your stomach and had to run off to the bathroom before you exploded, then you have certainly experienced something that most people have on at least one occasion. Maybe you have had the cramps that signal you really need to go "Number 2," but then you find that you sit on the toilet waiting and waiting just to find out that in actual fact you are constipated. Most people experience being gassy, bloated, constipated, having diarrhea, and many other digestive annoyances, at least from time to time, but what if you had that happen to you every day? If that is something you experience, and you consider that there could be a plethora of other related symptoms, then you could be a victim of conditions which are known by some as Leaky Gut Syndrome, Candida Overgrowth or Irritable Bowel Syndrome (often known as IBS).

Leaky Gut Syndrome is a health condition proposed by some health practitioners as being the root cause of a broad range of conditions, some of which can be long-term, including the likes of what is known as chronic fatigue syndrome, and multiple sclerosis (MS). The condition is described as a problem with the digestive tract, and it can also be known as "intestinal permeability," Proponents argue that it can cause a lot of discomfort and can be a particularly troublesome ailment. Assertion is made that different symptoms can range from diarrhea, to constipation, and even depression. Some even consider that having a "cloudy" mind is also associated with Leaky Gut. Some consider that there are many ways that Leaky Gut Syndrome may manifest itself within the body, and that the types of symptoms associated with Leaky Gut Syndrome are a result of conditions and medicines which cause intestinal permeability, which allows for germs, toxins and other substances to make their way into the bloodstream, triggering a reaction from the body's immune system.

Some proponents would argue that medical practice has not quite caught up to the serious, widespread ailment of Leaky Gut .However others in the medical profession, whilst considering that a leaky gut can indeed be caused by certain medications and conditions, take the view that there is not enough evidence to give widespread credence to the theory that significant problems can indeed be caused by a porous bowel.

In any case of this kind, it is important to be availed of as much information as possible – against which you can seek to make your own judgment. Of course, it stands to reason that it is highly recommended that you see a doctor before following any of the advice or suggestions you may find here, but there can be occasions where symptoms you may be experiencing can take a while to get to the bottom of, perhaps with repeat visits to the doctor to try to ascertain what really is ailing you.

If you experience many of the symptoms discussed in this book, then there are ways to try to improve resilience of your wider digestive and associated systems - helping yourself get better and feel better without necessarily having to have recourse to medical interventions – it makes sense to try and build as robust a system as possible. Often, it is our poor lifestyle choices which can contribute to our conditions, and therefore it is important to do for ourselves what we can before putting the responsibility of treatment on a doctor. Bear in mind too that such conditions can also have an impact on those around you – so it is in your, and their, best interests, that you seek to do what you can about your issues while you can. Much of the advice here can help you to build a resilient system and so be better placed to prevent those conditions such as Leaky Gut Syndrome.

Of course, taking control in such a situation does require a degree of self-help, but by dint of the fact that in reading this book, then it is clear that you are already trying to take control - you are already well placed to try and develop as tight and robust a system as you can – there are many routes to this, and we will try to help explain these. Of course there are no guarantees that these actions will actively support your digestive system in and of itself, but it does stand to reason that the healthier you are in body and mind, then the better chance there is of all of the systems in your body working together as they should – with the resultant sense of wellbeing for you.

Amongst all of the things that we have control over for our bodies and health, diet is arguably the most important, and it is considered by proponents that it greatly affects the chances and consequences of developing Leaky Gut Syndrome. There are other associated methods and measures we can consider, including the use of supplements and relieving stress, which can positively impact Leaky Gut Syndrome symptoms (as well as being good for wider health, wellbeing and mood. It will not be a surprise that if we consider diet, we'll also look at the impact exercise can have on building a more resilient system – how we take energy into our body, and the work we do to expend energy can have wider implications for how we function more generally.

It stands to reason that no one would willingly choose to live with such an ailment, so if you feel that you are experiencing the condition known as Leaky Gut Syndrome, then we hope that you feel this book can aid you in trying to understand the condition, and what you can do to try and get a degree of control over your digestive system.

Whilst the focus of this book is on Leaky Gut Syndrome, there are a couple of other issues which we thought were worthy of consideration – to try and give you a slightly wider picture – this means that we will consider conditions known as Candida Overgrowth Syndrome, and Irritable Bowel Syndrome (IBS).

Candida Overgrowth Syndrome is considered by some to be one of the many potential causes of Leaky Gut Syndrome, and is common enough that we thought an overview of it should be presented in this book. Left untreated, it is considered that it can lead to other problems, and again, the importance of having as resilient an underlying system as possible is paramount.

Irritable Bowel Syndrome, or IBS, while not life threatening in itself, is often painful and can be debilitating. Its sufferers often miss work or are unable to contribute to domestic life as they would like, and on occasion find that they cannot enjoy even the simple pleasures of life. They often suffer emotionally, and depression amongst sufferers can be an issue. We explore this a little, to try and give you an idea of what the condition is, the symptoms associated with it, and positive steps that you can take to try to manage the condition. Oftentimes the suggestions made align with others elsewhere in this book – no surprise really – it is the case that the basics of diet, exercise and managing stress levels are important for all our digestive related activities – and of course underpin our wider health too.

In this book, you will find out how to identify whether or not you may have Leaky Gut Syndrome, we will consider the other conditions mentioned above, and what you can do to help yourself if you believe you're afflicted with these. We will consider the role exercise can play in contributing to your overall wellbeing, and in considering diet, we offer some practical support by setting out some simple meal plans that will give you terrific and delicious ways to rid your body of harmful substances. If you want to learn how to use diet and other methods to calm and ease some of your digestive issues, then please take the time, and read on. By picking up this book, you have taken the first step – it is to be hoped that the information here can help you to take control. If that sounds good to you, and we hope it does, then let us see what happens next.

CHAPTER 1: WHAT IS DIGESTION?

As surprising as it sounds, many people do not understand the basics of the digestive system in their own bodies. Perhaps this is no surprise – it is part of our bodily function that the vast majority of us take for granted. Nonetheless it is a fundamental part of how our body works, and for this reason, we are going to include a brief description of what the digestive system is and how it works.

Digestion is effectively a process by which food is broken down into small parts that can be used by our bodies as fuel, creating the energy we need in order to function. This is accomplished by a number of different organs and glands which help our bodies to process food in this way. Food, when first eaten, is not in a state that we can easily convert to energy, so we have to break it down into parts small and soluble enough for us to turn into energy, and then we have to get rid of the waste products that are left over.

Almost all of the organs used in the digestive process, such as the stomach and the intestines, are shaped like tubes. Their functions are to move food through our bodies, and they often do this through series of muscular contractions. In fact, the entire digestive system is little more than a very long, undulating tube that goes all the way from your mouth to your rectum. Of course that is a very simplistic description and we will go into more depth, but in essence it is true – of course there are many glands, organs and other factors which combine to make sure everything works just as it should along the digestive tract. For example the pancreas and liver are important in helping to produce some of the chemicals used in the process of digestion, as well as ensuring a degree of balance in your system to ensure you are getting all the energy you need from food and drink that you take on board.

Of course the entire process starts when you put a bite of food into your mouth and start chewing. This starts the process of breaking the food down by grinding it into smaller pieces with the teeth, and this is aided by the salivary enzymes. These chemicals dissolve some of the starches and other nutrients so that they can be further processed by the stomach and intestines.

Once the food is chewed, you swallow it, and the partially processed food goes into your oesophagus. This is the long tube that goes from your mouth down to your stomach. Using muscle movements that are similar to waves moving down the length of the oesophagus, a motion that is known as peristalsis, it carries food down the throat and all the way to the stomach. Peristalsis, incidentally, is what makes it possible for us to eat and drink, even if we happen to be hanging upside-down at the time.

When the food gets to the stomach, which is a fairly good sized, bag-like organ, it is mixed with a powerful acid. Partly digested food that goes into the stomach and mixes with the acids there is known as chyme.

Once the stomach has provided the balanced environment for its stage of the digestive process, the food then goes into the duodenum, which is the very first section of the small intestine. From there, it moves into the jejunum, and finally it goes into the ileum, which is the last segment of your small intestine. You don't really need to know the detail of everything going on in each of these areas – but it is useful to have a general overview of what is going on down there!

While in your small intestine, bile, which comes from your liver and is kept in your gall bladder until it is needed, along with other enzymes that actually come directly from the inner lining of your small intestine begin to aid the breakdown of the food you've eaten.

Once the small intestine is done with it, the food then moves on to the large intestine. There, a portion of the water and other nutrients called electrolytes are taken from and moved to other parts of the body where they are needed. There are a lot of bacteria that actually live in your large intestine to help it during the digestion process.

The first section of your large intestine is called the cecum, and this is where the appendix is connected. After passing through this part, the food moves up through another part called the ascending colon. It moves across your body via the transverse colon, the part of your large intestine that goes across the top of the intestinal area, and then down again through your descending colon, and finally reaches the end of the line in your sigmoid colon. What's left over is then passed out through the rectum as waste.

There are many diseases, conditions and problems that can affect the digestion, and this book covers some of them. Its purpose is to give you, the reader, a better understanding of what goes on in your gut, and what might be going wrong in it. It is also hoped that you can use this basic understanding as a jumping off point to consider more about how your underlying systems operate – and so seek to build a more resilient you.

CHAPTER 2: WHAT IS LEAKY GUT SYNDROME?

If you have digestive issues, with symptoms that include gas, bloating, food sensitivities, cramps, and aches and pains, you could quite possibly have Leaky Gut Syndrome. However, digestive problems alone do not mean you have Leaky Gut, nor are the symptoms of Leaky Gut Syndrome purely digestive. "Leaky Gut Syndrome" (LGS) is a non-medical term for an ailment of the intestinal lining.

It is known that there is a single layer of cells which line the bowel – this is known as the mucosal barrier, that is it is the barrier between the inside of the gut and the rest of the body – it stands to reason that this lining is incredibly important for the normal functioning of the body. The barrier is very efficient at absorbing the nutrients contained in the food and drink we consume – but it is equally adept at stopping larger molecules and germs from passing from the bowel into the bloodstream – a situation which can lead to a wide variety of symptoms.

It is considered that, in certain situations, this key barrier can indeed become less effective, and so is sometimes described as "leaky" – in and of itself, this is not considered sufficient to cause particularly serious problems –though it does mean that it is more important than ever to try and eat and drink the right things (as well as being aware of what else can cause irritation of the lining of the bowel – such things include alcohol, aspirin and some anti-inflammatory medicines – this is one of the reasons it is suggested that anti-inflammatory drugs are taken whilst having something to eat). It is considered though, that irritant substances such as those mentioned above will rarely cause any issue more than a short lived inflammation of a certain part of the bowel (though it could be that inflammation is bad enough to cause, for example, ulcers in the bowel). Often the simple removal of a certain substance from a diet will be enough to cause the symptoms to improve relatively quickly.

There are other conditions, and also some treatments for other issues, which can cause damages to the bowel lining. These include:

- Coeliac disease

- Chronic kidney disease

- Inflammatory bowel diseases – for example Crohn's disease

- Intestinal infections – these can include food poisoning, salmonella, giardiasis and norovirus

- Medicines used for chemotherapy

- Abdominal radiotherapy

- HIV/AIDS

- Cystic fibrosis

- Type 1 diabetes

- Sepsis

- Complications from surgery

- Immunosuppresants

So, as we have considered, it is thought that if you have this condition, it means that your intestinal walls are more permeable than normal – this means that the bowel can allow too much to pass through the lining and into the bloodstream, as well as failing to absorb nutrients and lipids correctly as your body digests what you eat or drink. This can cause an unhealthy imbalance of bacteria in your body, as well as a change in the balance in the blood stream, as particles are allowed to pass into the body that would not ordinarily be there.

Unfortunately, there is much research left to be done on the digestive system and the intestines especially, and this means it can sometimes be difficult to be too precise.

Proponents of Leaky Gut Syndrome consider that the bowel lining itself can become irritated and so leaky due a wider range of factors than some of those we have outlined above. They assert that this can happen as a result when there is too much yeast or certain bacteria in the bowel, when a poor diet is undertaken or where there is an overuse of antibiotics in treatment of certain conditions. Proponents are considered to take the view that food particles which have not been fully digested, toxins and germs can get through the leaky gut (much as we have already described) and this in turn can cause the immune system to kick in, leading to inflammation in other parts of the body, as well as potentially leading to other ailments and conditions, which it is considered can include:

- Autism

- Skin conditions, for example excema

- Asthma

- Lupus, rheumatoid arthritis and multiple sclerosis (MS)

- Tiredness and chronic fatigue syndrome

- Migraine

- Food allergies.

Because of the slightly indeterminate range of symptoms which can be associated with Leaky Gut Syndrome, and the wide range of potential underlying factors, it is perhaps no surprise that many medical practitioners are reluctant to nail their colours to the mast on an issue which it is generally accepted does require more research – this means that doctors are unlikely to directly associate the symptoms and conditions described above as being caused by having a leaky gut. It is the case that it can be non-medically trained practitioners who take a more holistic view of the body that seek to make the case around Leaky Gut Syndrome. Of course many of the actions which they propose can be taken in relation to the condition are good for other reasons in and of themselves – in that they can help to build a more robust system – and that is good for a variety of reasons – related to mental as well as physical health and wellbeing.

Noticing your stomach and its reactions to foods is an important step in recognizing the symptoms of Leaky Gut Syndrome – but this is an area where, again, you can take an element of control by beginning to note down when symptoms seem to affect you, and what those symptoms are.

Unfortunately, in today's medical practice, most doctors are extremely busy and this means that they simply do not have the time available to actually try to find underlying causes for many conditions, and this can mean that their armory is more limited than even they might like, and this can lead to them simply prescribing this or that medication based on symptomatic data (maybe from one visit) only, without further examining any other factors. This is one reason why some people take the view that you might want to consider, as well as taking medical advice, seeing if you can find a practitioner whose diagnostic techniques and treatments are holistic in nature – but this approach does not mean that you can advocate responsibility either. Earlier we explored the types of symptoms associated with the conditions we are discussing in this book – you can be empowered, now you know what they are, to consider yourself whether these may be applicable to you, and so you can help with an element of self diagnosis. Of course some of the symptoms may be so severe that you need to ascertain whether you need a degree of emergency or at least quick medical assistance. However, it may be that have some of the less severe symptoms – maybe you experience them from time to time, rather than all at once – if this is the case, try and take some time to think about when you feel these symptoms. You might find that in doing this you struggle to recollect when such symptoms have affected you – if this is the case then you might want to think about considering whether you could pull together some sort of symptom calendar – if you can get something that works for you – whether this is paper or electronic based, then you might quickly start to be able to build up a wider picture of when particular symptoms are an issue – and when they appear together as well. All of this type of information will be useful for your doctor, and it also allows you to take on an element of control.

Many symptoms are also endured with a variety of other conditions, so it's best to seek diagnosis from a doctor. If you notice that you are often bloated and gassy with frequent stomach cramps, this is a sign that you could have Leaky Gut Syndrome. Other symptoms can include diarrhea or constipation, especially when eating certain types of foods, and aches and pains within the abdomen. Chrohn's and Celiac diseases also share some of these symptoms, so it is wise to consult a medical professional if you have any of these physical symptoms for more than a day or two. Extreme fatigue and body rashes can also be a result of too many toxins getting into the bloodstream through the intestines. It is thought by proponents that Leaky Gut Syndrome can even lead to acne, weight gain, headaches, and thyroid problems. It may be that you would wish to try and keep a diary to keep track of when certain symptoms show themselves.

Not only physical symptoms and causes are suspect. Depression and anxiety are suspected to sometimes be an effect of Leaky Gut Syndrome. This relates to the fact that the condition is not only physically uncomfortable, but can be embarrassing and inhibiting – with associated mental effects. An individual who has frequent diarrhea, for example, may be too embarrassed to stay at friends' houses for extended periods of time. Since there are both physical and mental causes and effects to Leaky Gut Syndrome, it is recommended to see both a doctor and a therapist when you suspect Leaky Guy Syndrome is having any effect upon your life. There are many things you can do to help yourself as well, and we will go over some of the best ways to deal with Leaky Gut Syndrome.

CHAPTER 3: CANDIDA

:Candida, a yeast type fungus, is something all of us have within us, though usually very little, living in our mouths and intestines. When it's functioning properly, it is considered that it aids in the absorption of nutrients and in digestion. Some people assert that something called Candida Overgrowth can be a serious medical condition that can have long lasting effects. Mainstream medical websites don't make much reference to this condition, and indeed don't make much reference to candida as it might appear in the gut, but the condition is referenced by holistic practitioners. As it is mentioned in some literature, it was thought prudent to include some reference in this book, together with views on how the condition can be managed.

The theory from proponents goes that when candida begins growing too rapidly, it can literally break through the intestinal wall and get into your bloodstream, allowing toxins to get into other parts of your body, and that this can cause Leaky Gut Syndrome. It is considered that when this happens, you can end up suffering from a number of different health problems, which can range from simple digestive problems to mild or even severe depression. Proponents assert that, generally, the healthy forms of bacteria that live in your gut tend keep candida levels where they belong. However, there are some things that can cause your natural candida population to begin growing out of control, such as:

- A diet that is rich in refined carbs and sugars

- Drinking excessive alcohol

- Using oral contraceptives

- A diet that is rich in foods that are fermented, like pickles and sauerkraut

- A stressful lifestyle

- Overuse of antibiotics leading to the loss of beneficial bacteria

Proponents of the condition assert that the symptoms of Candida Overgrowth can include things like:

1. Fungal infections of the skin and nails, like athlete's foot and toenail fungus

2. Chronic fatigue

3. Unexplained pains (fibromyalgia)

4. Diarrhea, bloating or constipation

4. Autoimmune diseases like Rheumatoid arthritis, Hashimoto's thyroiditis, Psoriasis, Multiple sclerosis, or Lupus

5. Poor memory, difficulty concentrating, trouble keeping focused, ADD or foggy thinking

6. Skin problems such as psoriasis, eczema, rashes or hives

7. Grumpiness, anxiety, mood swings or depression

8. Urinary tract infections, vaginal infections, rectal or vaginal itching

9. Unusually severe allergies

10. Cravings for sugar

DO YOU HAVE CANDIDA OVERGROWTH?

Those who take the view that the condition of candida overgrowth is a pertinent issue, and that it can be thought to lead to Leaky Gut Syndrome, set out a number of ways in which the condition can be diagnosed. These are as set out below:

Blood Test

Start by asking your doctor to check for candida antibodies, which are known as IgG, IgA, and IgM. This is a simple test, and high levels of these antibodies can indicate the presence of a candida overgrowth. Sometimes, however, these tests will turn out negative, even when other tests turn out positive.

Stool Test

This is usually the best way to determine if you might have this condition. The lab will want a stool sample, in order to check for the presence of candida in the colon or intestines, which will usually identify the species of yeast and what form of treatment will prove most effective. Be sure your doctor requests a stool test for candida.

Organix Dysbiosis

This is a urine test that looks for particular waste products of candida, which goes by the name of D-Arabinitol. A high level of this substance in your urine is indicative of candida overgrowth, and whether it may be present in your small intestine.

Treatment

In order to treat candida successfully, proponents of the condition consider that you must do three things: stop the overgrowth; restore the friendly gut bacteria; and heal your intestines so that waste products stop entering your bloodstream.

It is considered that the first thing that must be done is to eliminate the overgrowth, and that this means putting yourself onto a low-carb diet.

Yeasts feed on sugars, so it's necessary to get rid of sugar in all forms. This means giving up candy, alcohol, dessert and anything made from flour (starches). Reduce your intake of complex carbohydrates, like bread, beans, fruits, grains, pasta and potatoes, as well. This will stop candida from growing and help it to die off. It is recommended, however, that before you begin to exclude things from your diet that you do consult with a doctor for their advice.

Proponents of the condition also consider that individuals should consider cutting out all of the (generally beneficial) fermented foods, because, while fermented foods do aid in feeding the friendly bacteria, the truth is that harmful bacteria can feed off of them as well.

Treating with diet alone is not sufficient, though, as it may take up to six months to get candida under control again. Proponents assert that your doctor will probably suggest that you use anti-fungal medications for at least a month – this underlines that for gut related conditions, it is very important to keep your doctor in the loop – especially when making decisions around changing diet (and exercise regimes too).

If you're determined to treat yourself, and this is not advised, then proponents consider that you should look for what is known as a caprylic acid supplement. Caprylic acid is derived from coconut oil; it is thought to act by perforating the yeast cell wall, killing it.

More generally, there are actions which can be taken to try and rebuild the healthy bacteria that normally prevent candida from growing out of control. To do this, it is thought that an individual should take from 25,000,000,000 to 100,000,000,000 units of a good probiotic daily, in order to reduce the levels of candida and to rebuild the proper level of healthy bacteria.

It is then thought that there should be a related plan of action to begin to heal your gut. Get rid of foods that are likely to injure your gastro-intestinal tract, and start eating foods that help it to heal. This will stop candida doing its damage to your body, and those who follow the theory assert that this can drastically improve overall health.

CHAPTER 4: IRRITABLE BOWEL SYNDROME (IBS)

Irritable bowel syndrome (IBS) is a condition which is more recognised than the candida issue described above – it is better studied, and recognised by the medical profession, although it is still considered to be quite a wide-ranging condition – that is, that the symptoms which underlie it can be general and quite vague – and again this is the sort of condition where a degree of self-monitoring – of symptoms and diet, and how they interact – can go a long way to helping your doctor understand what is going on, and make the most appropriate decisions for your particular scenario. Irritable Bowel Syndrome, then, is usually identified by its symptoms, which are most commonly any kind of chronic or persistent pain in the abdomen, usually accompanied by bloating and changes in your bowel habits. It may be that you may suffer regular diarrhea or constipation, but they can alternate, so that you may be constipated one day, and afraid to get too far from the bathroom the next day. Of course it stands to reason that the symptoms vary between individuals, and of course some people will find that they have far more discomfort from the Syndrome than other people. It is also the case that the range of how long symptoms will last for will vary from person to person – maybe lasting a few days, or perhaps continuing for a few months at a time. It is also the case that there can be certain things which can set the condition off - these can include certain foods, or if you have been experiencing a particular stressful situation. Another factor is that you may find that going to the toilet and opening your bowels can ease certain symptoms of Irritable Bowel Syndrome.

It is considered that there is no known specific cause of Irritable Bowel Syndrome, however most doctors would assert that it relates to an increased sensitivity of the gut, and directly related to that issues with the digestion of food – this might show itself with food taking too long or too short a time to go through your gut, where the squeezing and relaxing of the muscles in your intestine do not operate in the rhythm that they should, leading to pain of one kind or another – and where it moves through the gut too fast, then it can lead to diarrhea, whilst if it moves through too slowly, then it leads to constipation (based on the premise that your body is absorbing too much water and this in turn leads to stools being hard, and so more difficult to pass. Some would assert that it does appear to be the case that it usually shows up after an infection or a particularly stressful period in your life. It does seem to affect up to one in five people at some stage in their life, and it is considered that it would usually begin to show itself as a condition at some point between the ages of 20 and 30 years old. It affects almost twice as many women as men, and whilst the condition can be lifelong, it can be managed, and indeed it may improve over several years.

It is also the case that some take the view that the root cause of Irritable Bowel Syndrome is down to a form of miscommunication between the brain and the intestines, that is the signals that travel back and forth to regulate what is going on in the gut are interrupted in some way. This can mean that the signals which tell someone with a normal functioning system whether they are hungry or full, for example, do not work properly, and this can mean that something which might cause mild discomfort for one person, can be painful for someone with Irritable Bowel Syndrome.

It is also the case that certain particular foodstuffs can trigger cases or bouts of Irritable Bowel Syndrome. It will not be much of a surprise to hear that these types of food and drink include fried food, or food with a lot of fat in it, alcohol, carbonated beverages, processed foods, and drinks which contain caffeine. Some people ned to watch out for chocolate too (though you can even get probiotic chocolate these days. As we consider elsewhere in this book, a really good idea is to try and keep a food diary to help you and your doctor understand whether any of these triggers may be a factor for you. Do what you can to help understand your own position, and that makes it easier for the doctors who will be trying to help you.

A doctor may diagnose you with Irritable Bowel Syndrome just from a review of your symptoms, as long as there are not additional indicators of a potentially more serious problem. If you have sudden unexplained weight loss, if there is blood in your stool, if you are showing any sign of an intestinal infection to perhaps colitis, then it's possible your doctor may order some tests to rule out anything more severe. The problem is that there are not specific tests for Irritable Bowel Syndrome, so what they do is test for the more serious conditions, and if they are not found, then it's probably Irritable Bowel Syndrome.

Then there's the fact that there are several diseases that may show the same types of symptoms, such as celiac disease, giardiasis and Leaky Gut Syndrome. Of course it is for your doctor to be able to draw the distinction.

The normal procedure for managing Irritable Bowel Syndrome is to treat the symptoms. This usually means making changes to your diet, reducing levels of stress and taking exercise – of course all of these things have an interplay between each other – some exercises such as yoga may also in and of themselves also help reduce stress levels. As regards diet, for Irritable Bowel Syndrome, some people find that taking regular probiotic products can help to ease symptoms – again, best to do this as part of a wider food diary to see if they make a difference for you. It is recommended that you would need to try probiotics for around four weeks to consider any discernible difference – of course you would not wait that long if you had more severe symptoms. In addition, it is recommended d that people with Irritable Bowel Syndrome learn more about fiber, and try to modify their intake. There are two types of fiber, soluble (which can be digested) and insoluble (which the body cannot digest). Examples of foods which contain soluble fiber include root vegetables, fruit, rye, barley and oats. Insoluble fiber containing foodstuffs include wholegrain bread, cereals and bran. Whilst you may get a mix of symptoms, if you tend to have diarrhea, then try to cut down on the insoluble fiber you eat, whilst if constipation is the bigger issue, then try to increase the amount of soluble fiber in your diet (together with ensuring you are having adequate hydration from the right sources – i.e. water!).

Some forms of medication are also available to help manage the symptoms of Irritable Bowel Syndrome – these include some which can help reduce the pain, others which ease constipation, some which help with diarrhea, and even low doses of anti-depressants which are used to reduce cramping for suffers of Irritable Bowel Syndrome. Of course it is for your doctor to make the judgment as to what is best for your particular scenario.

Irritable Bowel Syndrome, despite the fact that it is often painful and wears on the person suffering from it, is not a dangerous condition in and of itself. However, many people are unable to function normally while suffering its effects, and it can interfere with enjoying many of the normal pleasures of life, so there is a definite toll on the mental and emotional well being of the sufferer. People with Irritable Bowel Syndrome can be known to suffer from anxiety and depression, and these mental aspects are just as important to be aware of as the physical complaints at the root of the problem. Do seek support – many people suffer from Irritable Bowel Syndrome, and you are not on your own.

Remember that the most common symptoms of Irritable Bowel Syndrome show up as abdominal pain, usually with frequent constipation or diarrhea. In many cases, there will have been a recent alteration of your bowel habits, around the time it sets in. You may feel like you have to go right now, or like you didn't manage to get everything out when you did go. Sometimes, just managing to have a bowel movement will make the pain go away, but if your situation is ongoing or you feel it is more sever, then of course, your doctor is the next call to make.

CHAPTER 5: HOW TO USE DIET TO BUILD A MORE RESILIENT DIGESTIVE SYSTEM

We have talked already about the importance of diet – it stands to reason that the way energy is taken into our body's systems is of critical importance. The nutrient and energy balance of the food and drink we take on board is fundamental to how well our mind and body can function – but that does not mean that it is easy making the right decisions as to how to go about that. This section of the book seeks to introduce the concept of why diet is so important in trying to help regulate a well working digestive system – all with a view to easing you on the way to having the best balanced system you can have, in order to build wider resilience – in turn reducing the chances of developing particular conditions, or helping to reduce the impact of existing conditions. You are what you eat is a maxim you may have heard many times, but it really does stand to reason – we often try to remove ourselves a little from the decisions we make on what to eat, but they really are critically important. One thing to say, though, is that your diet is absolutely the number one thing that you are able to control. You make decisions on what to eat or drink every single day, and not only that, but many times each and every day – you are in control, and that is the first important lesson to take on board.

Related to this, one of the best things you can to begin, is to think about starting to keep a food diary – of course this could link in with the work you might already be doing in relation to symptoms, and could furthermore be used to detail other things which we will talk about shortly, for example relating to exercise, and even how you feel – if you can manage to detail all of these things together, then it becomes much easier to begin to spot patterns. Why don't you try it for a while, and see what results? There really is nothing to lose, and you might find that you begin to develop a really useful emerging picture of yourself that you hadn't particularly appreciated.

Primarily though, those who are proponents of the theory of Leaky Gut Syndrome make the case that in order to take on an element of control, you must first regulate what you put through your digestive system. This means that it is imperative when dealing with digestive issues to not only be aware of what you're eating, but to also eat things that soothe and aid Leaky Gut Syndrome rather than things that will aggravate the problem. So then, how do you know what will soothe and what will aggravate? That is a great question, and it will be clarified here shortly.

The first thing you're going to need to do is to cleanse your body of all the toxins and bacteria that may have been overloading your system. To do this, you will need a 14-21 day detox regime. This is only two to three weeks, and I can promise you it's not as difficult as you may be thinking. Dread for detoxing your body is only going to make things difficult for yourself. Instead of filling your mind with dread and nervous anxiety, get excited about the fact that you are taking genuinely constructive steps toward doing something important to help your body and to make yourself feel better. Also, understand that giving yourself a good detox does not have to mean that you can eat nothing but lettuce and lemon water, or that you're being deprived of taste for a couple of weeks. Even during detox, you can make delicious foods that will be satisfying.

Before starting your detox, you will be allowed one full day to eat as much of whatever you want. This is in order to satisfy any cravings you may have before getting started, as well as letting you feel how eating all the junk you want makes your body react. Notice how you feel immediately after eating, a couple of hours after eating, the night after you've eaten, and in the morning the next day.

It's very likely that those with Leaky Gut Syndrome will experience several symptoms during these times. You may want to take notes or make some sort of record of how you feel before starting your detox. This way, you will be able to compare how good detoxing makes your body feel and recognize how poor food choices can affect your body, making you feel bloated or gassy, or even causing you to have to run for the bathroom every few moments—even if sometimes you find you can't go, once you get there.

Fair warning: the detox that we're going to use, described below, is going to sound hard. It involves eating in a way that you're likely not used to, and not eating things that you may really enjoy. Remember that it is crucial to do a detox and stick to it in order to cleanse the body of the overload of toxins and harmful bacteria causing Leaky Gut Syndrome symptoms.

The good news is that you can eat as many of these things as you like: fruit, vegetables, nuts, seeds, beans, legumes, extra virgin olive oil, and tea. The hard part may be cutting out alcohol, dairy, gluten, grains, meats, sugar and artificial sweeteners. You may use Stevia if you find it necessary. Tiny amounts of honey are also permitted.

While this vegan detox may sound difficult to implement into your life, it's not that hard, and can be accomplished easily, especially for just two weeks. Recipes and meal plans will be included later in this book in order to make it even easier for you to follow this two-week detox schedule.

After doing a complete detox and sticking to it for two weeks, you can slowly begin to add in foods that were cut out. It's recommended to add one new food to your detox diet per week, in order to monitor the effects that such food may have on your body. For example, after detoxing for two weeks, you will continue to eat vegan, gluten- and dairy-free, but for the first week after, you may want to add cheese. This is fine, as long as you notice how the cheese affects your body and digestive system. If you find that, after detoxing, you felt great, but adding cheese brings on symptoms of Leaky Gut Syndrome, you will want to switch to non-dairy cheeses. There are plenty to choose from, since vegan and vegetarian diets have become more popular over the last couple of decades.

Incidentally, don't panic; this doesn't mean you need to become a vegetarian for the rest of your life. On the contrary; your body was designed to receive a substantial part of its nutrients from meats, including those that come from both proteins and fats. Meats can be added back into your diet after the detox, but be wise enough to do so lowly, and keep a record of how your body reacts to each item you bring back into your diet. That way, you can spot trouble causing foods as they begin to affect you, and adjust your diet as needed.

In addition to detoxing and diet adjustment, there are some other things you can do to ease Leaky Gut Syndrome. For example, soothing herbs can greatly help ease symptoms. Some of these herbs and plants to include in teas or in your food are: dandelion root, peppermint, cumin, licorice root, turmeric, and ginger. It's also important to get plenty of fiber, which can be supplemented with: flax seed, oats, cinnamon, rosemary, basil, and parsley. Fermented raw vegetables, such as sauerkraut, carrots, beets, radishes, and turnips, can greatly help with intestinal issues and are recommended to be eaten frequently. Glutamine, zinc, and probiotics have also shown to help ease symptoms of Leaky Gut Syndrome.

Hydration

A further factor to bear in mind in this diet is hydration – proper levels of hydration are absolutely critical to all our bodily functions – not least cognitive ability and digestive function. Without proper hydration, the body loses energy very quickly and it's unlikely to survive more than three days without any water. Drinking enough water is vital to having a healthy body. Water makes up the largest percent of what our bodies are made of, so it makes sense that we should consume a good amount of it in order to stay healthy. If you are to be eating properly, then you must also be drinking properly.

Directly related to this is what you may be drinking that is acting to dehydrate you – traditional tea, coffee and alcohol all acts to dehydrate – but there are so many alternatives on the market that you do not need to have to give up your routine of a hot drink at certain times of the day, and you can try to lessen your alcohol intake by replacing with soft drink options. Perhaps get yourself a soft drink cocktail book and see if you can make things a bit more interesting at home. Try also to have water with you when you leave the home – it is important to stay hydrated throughout the day and you may find it benefits you in relation to staying concentrated – often an issue even when in a sedentary occupation, where you may be looking at a computer screen or papers through the day.

Of course if you are exercising (as we suggest is also important) then there will be an additional need to ensure you are taking on board enough water.

CHAPTER 6: RECIPES FOR DETOX

We mentioned earlier that it is one thing to say you want to take on a detox diet, but it is something else to actually make it happen in a successful manner. To that end we have chosen to provide a variety of dietary suggestions toy allow you to take the first steps. There are many more recipe options available which might do the job for you, but those given here should allow you to make a good start – and you can then improvise as you see fit.

In order to follow a detox meal plan, or any meal plan for that matter, it's important to know how and what to prepare for yourself during the scheduled diet. For this reason, there are several recipes that are safe for detox dieting included here. While there are many more things you can prepare to eat, these recipes should give you a great starting point for following your detox plans with easy and delicious foods to prepare.

It is worth thinking about how you can monitor what you are eating – why don't you start right now by beginning to take a note of what you are actually eating – and you can start to plan some of the suggestions below into what you are going to eat next. This also means that you are able to look back and see what progress you have made over time. It also means that you can start to plan your food shops based on what you need for the recipes we suggest – it might be that some of the ingredients have been hiding at the back of your cupboard for a while anyway, but it is also the case that you could consider stocking up on some staples – that might be easier if you have access to online shopping where you can keep a close eye on what you are buying, but if this isn't an option for you, try to take a tight list of what you need to the store – and try not to be sucked in by the inevitable promotions which will face you on arrival!

All that said then, here are a few ideas to get you started. Remember, some of these options may include things which you maybe think you are not too keen on, but the combinations with other foodstuffs can lead to different textures and tastes, and you may find that you begin to change your mind – in any case, there really is nothing to lose.

RECIPES

SWEET SNACKS

Banana Bars

2 Bananas

1 Cup Almond Butter

Nuts/Dried fruit/Flax Seeds/Other (optional)

Mash bananas and mix with almond butter until well blended. Add nuts, dried fruits, or other allowed ingredients to customize your bars. Bake at 350 degrees for around 20 minutes and allow to cool completely before eating.

Banana Pudding

Banana

Almond Butter (optional)

Almond Milk

Flax seeds

In a food processor or blender, mix banana with about half a cup of almond milk. Add 1 tsp flax seeds. Blend in almond or other nut butter if desired, about 1 tbsp. Allow to sit in the fridge for at least one hour before eating.

Cocoa Banana "Ice-Cream"

1 Banana, mashed

cocoa powder, to taste

stevia, to taste (optional)

Mix one mashed banana with stevia and cocoa powder. You may blend these together or use a food processor for best results. Freeze in a sealed container for 2-4 hours.

BREAKFASTS

Fruit Smoothie

Almond Milk

Banana

Frozen Berries

Water

In a blender, pour half a cup of almond milk and ¾ cup water. Slice banana and put into blender. Add frozen berries until they barely peek over the liquid. Add more water as needed. Blend until smoothed to desired consistency.

Overnight Oats

Almond Milk

Fruit of choice

Gluten-free Oats

½ tbsp Honey

Mix 1 cup oats with 2/3 cup almond milk. Add fruit and honey. Leave in refrigerator overnight in a mason jar or similar sealable container. Mix well in the morning before eating.

Veggie Scramble

2 eggs

Spinach

Tomato

Spices of your choice

Cooking spray

Mix eggs, spinach, and chopped tomato in a bowl. Spray a pan with cooking spray and pour bowl contents onto pan when hot. Cook until eggs are no longer runny.

LUNCHES

Garden Salad

Spinach

Carrots

Avocado

Cucumber

Onion

Broccoli

In a large bowl, mix desired amount of spinach, chopped or sliced carrots, chopped or sliced avocado, sliced cucumber, chopped onion, and chopped broccoli. Top with lemon and olive oil as dressing. Instead of dressing add black beans on top to make "Bean Salad".

Nachos

Vegetable Chips (ensure only ingredients are vegetables and oil)

Gluten-free vegan refried beans

Guacamole/Avocado

Create a bed of chips on a plate. Top with refried beans and guacamole or avocado. Eat warmed or cold.

Summer Salad

Cucumbers

Avocado

Tomato

Onion

Olives

Red Pepper

Pepperoncini Peppers

Olive Oil

Balsamic Vinegar

Chop and mix all ingredients in a bowl. Cover and leave in the refrigerator for at least one hour before consuming.

DINNERS

Cauliflower Rice

Cauliflower

Clove of garlic, minced

Lime, to taste

Cilantro, to taste

Olive Oil

Salt and Pepper, to taste

Using a grater or food processor, grate the cauliflower into rice-sized granules. Heat a tablespoon of oil in a skillet, and add minced garlic. Add grated cauliflower and cook 5-6 minutes, adding cilantro and lime. After cooking, you can add lettuce, tomato, beans, and avocado to create your own "burrito bowl".

"Spaghetti"

Spaghetti Squash

Olive Oil

Seasonings, to taste

Lemon/Olive oil/garlic OR tomato sauce

Cut spaghetti squash in half and drizzle with olive oil. Sprinkle on desired seasonings and bake cut-side-down at 400 degrees for about an hour. The squash should be very tender when finished. Allow squash to cool for a few minutes, then take a fork and scrape out the squash "noodles". Serve and cover with lemon juice, olive oil, and garlic or the spaghetti sauce of your choosing.

7-Bean Soup

7 Cans of different beans

Carrots and other desired vegetables

2 Cloves Garlic chopped

½ onion chopped

Seasonings, to taste

Mix seven types of canned beans into a crock pot. I like to use pinto, cannelloni, garbanzo, black-eyed, black beans, kidney beans, and navy beans, but you can use whatever you wish. Add largely chopped carrots, vegetables, garlic, and onion. Season to your desired taste and allow to cook on low setting for 8 hours. Alternate cans of beans for canned vegetables in order to make "Vegetable Soup".

Zucchini Boats

Zucchini

Garlic, chopped

Onion, chopped

Tomato sauce

Cut zucchini in half lengthwise. Scoop out middle part of zucchini, and mix with garlic, onion, and tomato sauce. Put mixture back into hollowed zucchini and bake at 350 for about twenty minutes.

Mushroom Soup:

Mushroom Bouillon

Chopped Mushrooms

Chopped Cauliflower

Minced Garlic

Chopped Onion

Seasonings, to taste

Mix ingredients in a crock pot and allow to cook on low setting for 8 hours.

Tip: Some Additional Recipes (Drawn from Public Domain Sources)

VEGETARIAN CHICKEN SALAD

Chopped protose, ½ pound.

Chopped celery, ⅔ cup.

Grated onion, 1 small teaspoonful.

Chopped nuttolene, ¼ pound.

Lemons, juice of 2.

Salt.

Mayonnaise, 2 tablespoonfuls.

Mix all together, adding mayonnaise dressing last. Serve on lettuce.

ALMOND SALAD

Olives, 18.

Celery, 1½ cups.

Blanched almonds, 1½ cups.

Salad dressing.

Lettuce.

Stone and chop the olives. Add the almonds chopped, also the celery cut fine. Mix with salad dressing and serve on lettuce.

NORMANDIE SALAD

Walnut meats, 1 cup.

French peas, 1 can.

Mayonnaise.

Lettuce.

Place walnut meats in scalding water about fifteen minutes, then remove the skins, and cut into pieces about size of a pea. Scald the French peas, and set aside for a while. Drain the water off the peas, and let them get cold; then mix with the walnuts. Pour mayonnaise dressing over all, and mix thoroughly. Serve on lettuce.

BRAZILIAN SALAD

Ripe strawberries, 1½ cups.

Fresh pineapple, cut in small cubes, 1½ cups.

Brazil nuts, blanched and thinly sliced, 12.

Lemon juice, 4 tablespoonfuls.

Lettuce.

Dressing, 1 spoonful.

Cut the strawberries and pineapples into small cubes, and add thinly-sliced Brazil nuts that have been marinated in lemon juice.

Arrange lettuce in rose-shape, and fill the crown with the above mixture, and cover with a spoonful of mayonnaise or golden salad dressing.

FRUIT SALAD

Apples, cut in half-inch cubes, 1 cup.

Bananas, cut in half-inch cubes, 1 cup.

Oranges, cut in half-inch cubes, 1 cup.

Mix all together and serve with golden salad dressing.

WALDORF SALAD

Apples, cut in dice, 1½ cups.

Lemon juice, ½ cup.

Lettuce.

Celery, cut in dice, 1½ cups.

Mayonnaise dressing.

Mix apples, celery, and lemon juice well together, and pour mayonnaise dressing over. Serve on lettuce.

In making Waldorf salad use only crisp, white, tart apples, and the tender, white heart of the celery. The celery should be cut a little smaller than the apples. Use only white mayonnaise.

Drain off the lemon juice before adding the dressing, or it will ruin the mayonnaise.

VEGETABLE BOUILLON

Vegetable soup stock, 2 quarts.

Cooked and strained tomatoes, 2 cups.

Bay leaves, 2.

Salt, 1 tablespoonful.

Onions, grated, medium size, 2.

Mix all the ingredients together, and let simmer slowly two or three hours. There should be about one quart of soup when done; strain, reheat, and serve.

NUT CHOWDER SOUP

Nuttolene or protose, ¼ pound.

Hard-boiled eggs, 3.

Browned onions, 3.

Sage, 1 teaspoonful.

Thyme, 1 teaspoonful.

Bay leaves, 2.

Salt, 1 tablespoonful.

Chop all together till fine, then add to strained boiling tomatoes, four cups; add boiling water, one cup; thicken with flour, one tablespoonful; reheat and serve.

NUT FRENCH SOUP

Vegetable soup stock, 1½ quarts.

Tomatoes, cooked, strained, 2 cups.

Sage, ¼ teaspoonful.

Browned flour, 1 tablespoonful rounded.

Onions, large, 1.

Bay leaves, 2.

Thyme, ½ teaspoonful.

Salt to taste.

Slice the onion and mix all the ingredients together, excepting the salt; boil slowly one hour; strain, reheat, salt, and serve. This soup requires plenty of salt to bring out the flavor.

MOCK CHICKEN SOUP

Butter, ¼ cup.

Onion, medium size, 1.

Celery stalks, 1.

Milk, 1¼ quarts.

One egg.

Flour, 2 tablespoonfuls.

Parsley, chopped fine, 1 teaspoonful.

Nuttolene, 3 tablespoonfuls.

Flour.

Put butter in saucepan with the onion, parsley, and celery; cook it to a golden brown color; add the flour and cook until brown, being careful not to scorch. Now add the milk boiling hot and stir briskly to prevent lumping. Add the nuttolene. Beat the egg with enough flour to make a stiff batter, but thin enough to pour; pour this into the boiling stock, stirring at the same time. This will appear as small dumplings in the soup. Let simmer twenty or thirty minutes; salt, and serve.

MOCK CHICKEN BROTH

Small white beans, 2 cups.

Small onion, 1.

Salt.

Hot water, 8 cups.

Celery salt.

Butter.

Wash, then stew the beans in hot water with the onion for three hours, stewing down to six cups; strain, and add a pinch of celery salt and a small piece of butter. Salt to taste. This broth may be served to the sick instead of beef tea.

PLAIN VEGETABLE SOUP

For soup stock.

Water, 6 cups.

Strained tomatoes, 2 cups.

Shave in fine shreds, add to soup stock, and cook moderately for two hours.

Carrot, 1.

Potato, 1.

Leek, 1.

Turnip, 1.

Onions, 2.

Celery stalk, 1.

Add a little sage and thyme. When done, run through puree sieve or colander, and add a little chopped parsley and salt to taste.

CHAPTER 7: 14 DAY DETOX PLAN + ONE WEEK AFTER

Of course you may have scanned the recipe list above, seen some things you like the look of, but feel as if you don't have time to factor them into a meal plan. We have tried to take make this a little easier by providing a template for a two week detox, followed by suggestions for the week after.

Of course, fourteen days, or two weeks, may seem overwhelming for many people to begin and stick to a detox diet. However, the plan is to show you how to do it easily, without feeling like you are starving or deprived of flavor. When you set out to start detoxing, it can be much easier to take it three days at a time.

After three days, congratulate and reward yourself for sticking to it—just don't reward yourself with foods!—and get ready for the next three days. This can be much more manageable, and less stressful for you, than taking on two whole weeks in one go. We've included 14 days worth of a meal plan for detoxing, as well as how you can incorporate new foods after your detox. While we hope these plans are useful and helpful to you, do not feel that you're somehow required to stick to it religiously. As long as you stay within the boundaries of what you can eat during your detox, have whatever strikes your fancy. In addition to the foods you eat, it is imperative to drink enough water and stay hydrated every day – we touched on this earlier, but it is absolutely imperative, and something you should try and build into your daily routines, not just looking for water when you find you are thirsty.

Meal:		Day Two:	Day Three:
Brea		Overnight Oats	Veggie Scramble
Lu	Salad	Nachos	Summer Salad
	ghetti"	Cauliflower Rice Bowl	7 Bean Soup
Snack	Hummus and carrots Unlimited Fruit/Veg	Banana Pudding Unlimited Fruit/Veg	Banana "Icecream" Unlimited Fruit/Veg

Meal:	Day Four:	Day Five:	Day Six:
Breakfast	Overnight Oats	Smoothie	Veggie Scramble
Lunch	Nachos	Summer Salad	Garden Salad
Dinner	Vegetable Soup	"Spaghetti"	Zucchini Boats
Snack	Nuts and dried fruit Unlimited Fruit/Veg	Hummus and carrots Unlimited Fruit/Veg	Banana Bars Unlimited Fruit/Veg

Meal:	Day Seven:	Day Eight:	Day Nine:
Breakfast	Fruit bowl	Overnight Oats	Smoothie
Lunch	Bean Salad	Nachos	Garden Salad
Dinner	Cauliflower Rice Bowl	7 Bean Soup	Mushroom Soup
Snack	Banana Pudding Unlimited Fruit/Veg	Nuts and Dried Fruit Unlimited Fruit/Veg	Banana "Icecream" Unlimited Fruit/Veg

Meal:	Day Ten:	Day Eleven:	Day Twelve:
Breakfast	Scrambled Eggs	Smoothie	Overnight Oats
Lunch	Nachos	Summer Salad	Garden Salad
Dinner	"Spaghetti"	Zucchini Boats	7 Bean Soup
Snack	Banana Bars Unlimited Fruit/Veg	Carrots and Hummus Unlimited Fruit/Veg	Banana Pudding Unlimited Fruit/Veg

Meal:	Day Thirteen:	Day Fourteen:

Breakfast	Veggie Scramble	Fruit Bowl
Lunch	Nachos	Garden Salad
Dinner	Cauliflower Rice Bowl	"Spaghetti"
Snack	Banana "Icecream" Unlimited Fruit/Veg	Cucumber with guacamole rolls Unlimited Fruit/Veg

WEEK AFTER DETOX:

Meal:	Day One:	Day Two:	Day Three:
Breakfast	Overnight Oats	Smoothie	Veggie Scramble with cheese
Lunch	Nachos	Summer Salad with feta cheese	Garden Salad
Dinner	Vegetable Soup	"Spaghetti"	Zucchini Boats, topped with cheese
Snack	Nuts and dried fruit, cheese stick Unlimited Fruit/Veg	Hummus and carrots, cheese stick Unlimited Fruit/Veg	Banana Bars Unlimited Fruit/Veg

Meal:	Day Four:	Day Five:	Day Six:
Breakfast	Scrambled Eggs	Smoothie	Overnight Oats
Lunch	Nachos with cheese	Summer Salad with feta cheese	Garden Salad
Dinner	"Spaghetti"	Zucchini Boats	7 Bean Soup, top with sprinkled cheese
Snack	Banana Bars Unlimited Fruit/Veg	Carrots and Hummus, cheese stick Unlimited Fruit/Veg	Banana Pudding Unlimited Fruit/Veg

Meal:	Day Seven:
Breakfast	Veggie Scramble with cheese
Lunch	Nachos
Dinner	Cauliflower Rice Bowl
Snack	Banana "Icecream" Unlimited Fruit/Veg

Tip: Remembering the Herbal Approach

It is important to remember that there is a particular set of foodstuffs which can not only enhance the taste of many recipes, but can also be considered as contributing their own health benefits. This means that it is fair to say that herbs are making a comeback. Once considered an outdated practice, herbalism is now seeing a huge revival, with millions of people taking advantage of the healing power of plants and flowers. It's not just for your hippie uncle, anymore! Out of the hundreds of thousands of different kinds of plants on the planet, we humans have identified over a hundred that have potent medicinal effects and have been using them to heal ourselves for centuries. Before modern medicine came along, it was plants that made up the majority of medical care, both for acute and chronic illnesses, but rest assured, nowadays we have a lot more regulation on the quality and use of such remedies, herbalists must be certified, products must be tested for safety and potency, and the cultivation practices are more sustainable than in eras past.

If you have ever walked through the aisles of a health food store, you will have no doubt noticed the shelves stacked high with herbal tinctures, pills, and powders. This can make it a little scary to take your chances with them, but trust me, with the right knowledge and direction, you can incorporate the power of plants into your health quest, and it's not as far out there as some might think.

For example, have you heard of Echinacea? Probably so, as it's a very popular immune support supplement. What about St. John's Wort? Perhaps you have, since lots of people use this herb for dealing with depression, and chances are you have used Ginseng, or know someone who has, as it's added to dozens of energy-boosting formulas used all over the world.

Many of us incorporate herbal remedies into our lives without even being aware of it, but if you truly want to heal yourself, you should consider adding specific plants and herbs to your supplement regimen. While interactions and side effects with pharmaceutical medications are commonplace, those with herbal supplements are generally few and far between, and if they do occur, they are typically very mild and very rarely life threatening. If you are concerned about this possibility, most drug interaction sites now include a variety of natural and herbal options that you can check for warnings. In addition, as we have already discussed, you can discuss such issues with your doctor.

In addition to the examples above, here are a few of the most widely-used plants in the herbal medicine realm, and what they're typically considered by proponents to be most useful for:

Garlic—cardiovascular issues, atherosclerosis, high cholesterol, high blood pressure, immune support (raw garlic is great at fighting colds/flus)

Gingko biloba—poor memory and concentration, aging-related cognitive decline, Alzheimer's disease

Feverfew—headaches (including migraines), menstrual cramps, general pain relief

Maca root—hormonal imbalances, low libido, fatigue, infertility

Evening primrose—PMS (both mood and cramping), hormonal imbalances, some cardiovascular disease

Lavender and Chamomile—insomnia, anxiety, ADHD, general stress relief

Goldenseal—immune support, antiseptic, soothing mucus membranes, anti-viral

Turmeric—arthritis, joint pain, fibromyalgia, aging related decline

Cinnamon—diabetes and pre-diabetes, blood sugar regulation, weight control, high cholesterol

Ginger—nausea, bloating, gas, stomach irritation, motion sickness, high blood pressure, arthritis, general pain relief

Basil—stress relief, adrenal fatigue, irritability, inhibits cancer growth

There are many great ways to utilize the power of herbs in your life, and it is considered by proponents that you can feel safe because you are using a 100% natural product which helps your body heal at the deepest level instead of simply masking symptoms – bear in mind what we have said about making sure you speak to your doctor if you are having symptoms thought to be associated with Leaky Gut Syndrome however. Most herbs are also available as pills, powders, liquids, topical creams/gels, teas, and tinctures. Find which versions you like the best and are the most likely to use on a regular basis, because like anything, consistency is key when recovering from illness! Herbs especially tend to have an added effect over time, so even if you don't feel immediately better, keep taking them—in a month or two you will have reached a whole new level of health and vitality.

If you have a serious condition that has been complicated to treat in the past, you may want to do your research on the types of herbs available to you and find a combination or "stack" that will give you the best benefit, but start with one at a time, so you can track your progress before adding in the next one. Consult with books, reputable websites, or even a certified herbalist or naturopath to discover the potential that plants can bring to your healing journey.

Tip: The Long Term Importance of Diet

We've already talked about the things you should avoid eating, and some that you should eat, but diet isn't just about a few things. It's time you take complete charge of your diet and complete responsibility for what you put into your body. To do so, you'll need to gain a good understanding of what a proper diet really is, and while that is beyond the scope of this book, nonetheless, here are some tips that will help.

What you choose to eat and drink can have a powerful effect on your state of health, and nutrition is only just starting to get the attention it deserves in the wellness community. Good nutrition, of course, is the foundation of any healing process, and has the ability to transform our bodies from the inside out. When our bodies are nourished and fed, we can experience healing on a deep level, even if we don't quite understand how it's happening yet. There is still plenty of research that needs to be done on foods and how they affect our bodies, but in the meantime we have enough to give us a good idea of how our bodies prefer to be fueled.

Now, there is a lot of confusing and conflicting information out there in the world of nutrition, and just a simple Google search will turn up thousands of books and blogs on the subject, each with their own opinions. We have to remember, however, that our bodies know best, and that we all have some ideas about what foods make us feel good and what foods don't. When you really think about how your body and mind responds to a satisfying, fresh, and healthy meal, this is you gently being guided to sound nutrition. This should not be confused, however, with the temporary high that certain foods give us. Candy, donuts, soda, and even buttery mashed potatoes can all send chemical signals to our brains that signal pleasure. This is a much different feeling than the deep, lasting feeling of well-being that healthy food provides.

If you are struggling with a problem like Leaky Gut Syndrome, your diet should be the first place you look to make changes. Depending on the seriousness of your condition, your body will require varying degrees of nourishment, and this includes macronutrients like protein, fat, and carbohydrate, as well as things like vitamins and minerals. The key is to get the most nutrition benefit when sitting down for a meal, meaning the more nutrients you can cram in, the better of you're likely to be. In some cases, such as with cancer and autoimmune diseases, additional supplements may be needed, because you simply cannot eat that many calories in a day. Look for high-quality multi-vitamins, amino acids, and other natural formulas and be sure to take the advice of your doctor.

Regardless of your health challenge, you should include lots of green leafy vegetables, cruciferous vegetables, good quality protein, healthy fats, and relatively few carbohydrates. Also, processed and packaged foods are generally a no-go, given the chemicals and other additives, and high sugar and sodium content. Eating as naturally as possible is a great way to make sure you are getting the nutrition you need; foods that can be found in nature, look like they do in nature, and come from a natural source are the best choices (e.g., a whole chicken vs. chicken nuggets).

You should not necessarily always be afraid of fat, as it is protective and nourishing for your cells, especially your nervous system, but your fat should come from natural sources like avocados, meat, fish, nuts, and coconut, as opposed to harmful refined and trans fats that are added to processed foods. Eating clean and satisfying fatty foods of the right type, and in appropriate quantities are unlikely to lead to heart disease! It is considered that it is actually the inflammation caused by high-sugar, highly processed, and otherwise altered foods that contribute to a disease state.

A little information on carbohydrates: unless you are an elite athlete, you actually do not need to consume very many carbohydrates in a day, though of course they have a part to play in a well-balanced diet. Furthermore, you can get carbs from totally natural sources like fruits, vegetables, sweet potatoes, and sweeteners like honey and maple syrup—no processed grains necessarily required! Many people actually have a low-grade inflammation reaction to grains, and it is especially bad in autoimmune diseases and gut-related illnesses, so finding replacements for those is a key step in allowing your body to heal.

Yes, it may take time to change your eating habits, especially if you are still stuck in the normal modern western diet, but it will be the biggest leap forward you can manage in terms of your health. When you concentrate on eating lots of fresh vegetables and fruits, healthy fats, organic meats, and including extra supplements if needed, you are giving your body the tools it needs to get well and stay well. Start swapping out the giant bowls of pasta for giant bowls of salad or sauteed veggies, and nix the nightly ice cream (dairy can also be an inflammatory trigger for some) in favor of fruit and dark chocolate, and see how you feel.

And remember, the foods you put into your body are just as powerful as any drug, especially when examining the diet over time. You have the choice today to stop poisoning your body and start nourishing it instead! And when you nourish your body, you will have better sleep, fewer aches and pains, and faster healing from whatever is bothering you.

CHAPTER 8: TREATMENT OF LEAKY GUT

While it is important to fix your diet and to do a detox when experiencing Leaky Gut Syndrome, it is not only a two week fix to complete health. While the 14 day detox will help to ease the symptoms and clear your body of harmful toxins, it takes more of an effort than that to completely help yourself to not only ease the symptoms, but to prevent and treat them. Proponents consider that there are many methods you can use in order to treat Leaky Gut Syndrome. These treatments include supplements, alternative treatments, and calming your digestive tract.

In addition, it is considered that you should avoid processed meats in any form since almost all of them contain antibiotics that are fed to the animals in an attempt to keep them healthier. The problem with this is that those antibiotics filter down to us, when we consume the meat, and this is, in the view of some, a major contributor to the so called "superbugs' that plague us today; germs we encounter get used to the many different kinds of antibiotics in our bodies and develop resistance to them, so that they no longer have the health benefits we have come to expect from them. It's important also to avoid taking too many antibiotics when sick, and to never take them when they're not actually needed. For example, the common cold is a viral infection rather than bacterial, so antibiotics are unnecessary and completely useless in combating it.

Instead, take your antibiotic regimen into your diet. Adding spices like garlic, red pepper, oregano, cinnamon, anise, sassafras and nutmeg will aid your immune system in fighting off infections naturally. Nutmeg, garlic and oregano, in particular, have been shown to be effective in fighting many bacterial infections, and some fungi. Using them in cooking may reduce their efficacy somewhat, but there are still many benefits, and most are also available as herbal supplements.

While staying away from antibiotic overload, it's also a good idea to cut out all unnecessary aspirin, ibuprofen, and other anti-inflammatory drugs (though don't do this without talking to your doctor if these have been prescribed to you for medical reasons). In addition, taking non-essential prescription drugs can have a negative effect on the digestive system, and it would be a great idea to talk to your doctor about any prescription drugs you are taking to find out if there are more natural methods to try. For example, turmeric is a great anti-inflammatory herb from the ginger family that can be taken as a supplement or added to food as a seasoning.

Another thing you can do long term in order to prevent symptoms of Leaky Gut Syndrome is to stay away from gluten products as much as possible. While many of the foods popular today contain gluten, the substance can create the permeability in the intestines that causes problems such as Leaky Gut Syndrome and other digestive ailments. Gluten products include anything made with wheat (most cereals, breads, pasta, pizza, snack foods, cookies and cakes, as well as many soups, gravies, sauces and condiments), corn, barley, rye and many other grains. Gluten intolerance is one of the most prevalent conditions affecting people today, even more than lactose intolerance, and it has even been linked by some to increasingly common conditions such as thyroid problems, obesity, diabetes type II, autism and more.

Some fermented foods are considered as a useful addition to a lifestyle that aims to rid the body of Leaky Gut Syndrome. Kefir is one product that is recommended. It's a fermented, cultured probiotic drink that contains many more good bacteria than cultured yogurt. It supports the digestive and immune systems, and can multiply the healthy bacteria within the intestines. Although kefir is often made from cow's milk, it is almost entirely lactose-free.

Umeboshi is another fermented food. These fermented plums, like other fermented foods, contain good bacteria and probiotic properties that can greatly affect the gut in a positive way.

Some great supplements to add to your daily routine can also help with Leaky Gut Syndrome symptoms and gut repair. L-Glutamine is one of these supplements. It is an amino acid, a building block of protein, which helps to repair the permeability of the gut that causes LGS. Another supplemental aid is Ultraimmune IgG, which contains an antibody that improves the immune functions of the digestive system and helps in reducing toxins and flushing waste from the body.

Aloe vera, coconut oil, and Omega-3's such as fish oil and krill oil are also helpful in helping to ease and fix the gut when experiencing Leaky Gut Syndrome. Aloe is helpful because it's one of the best natural detoxifying products you can get. Packed with vitamins and minerals, drinking aloe is a fantastic digestive aid that is incredibly healthy and good tasting. Coconut oil absorbs quickly and easily in the intestines, and can help nutrients be absorbed as well. It's also better for the digestive system than most other types of oils. Omega-3 supplements can reduce inflammation of the digestive tract, but also may cause diarrhea and other side effects, so use them at your own discretion.

Tip: Pay Attention to yourself!

The age of mindfulness has arrived. Finally the modern world is catching up on the wisdom that has been held by gurus and monks for centuries, and realizing that mental training has tremendous benefits. Numerous studies are being published every month about the metabolic and psychological effects of meditation and mindfulness training, and the health and wellness experts couldn't be more pleased. Thought it was once considered only a strictly spiritual and relaxation practice, meditation can now be found everywhere from classrooms to boardrooms.

Most people are aware that high stress can lead to many unfortunate consequences: reduced immune function, disrupted sleep patterns, and predisposition to disease to only name a few. Our age of chronic mental tension has precipitated an epidemic of sick and unhappy people, but luckily now we are beginning to understand, from a scientific standpoint, that we have the power to change that in only a few minutes per day. Meditation, when done correctly, can put our bodies in a state of relaxation, and this zone of calm is where the healing magic happens. You see, your body cannot heal itself when you are constantly stressed all the time, and running around like a rabbit from one deadline and meeting to the next. We were not designed to function this way, our modern age of "do it all and don't let them see you trying" is making us seriously sick.

When you are faced with a stressor, be that a huge work project, a screaming child, or even things like environmental pressures (e.g., a claustrophobe in a jammed subway car), your body goes into the "fight or flight" mode. Your organs kick into gear, churning out stress hormones, boosting your heart rate and blood pressure, halting digestion, and loads of other things. This is an age-old response from when our ancestors needed to act quickly in a threatening situation in order to survive and produce offspring. Sadly, while our daily stressors are not typically life threatening, our bodies still react in the same way, and this chronic stressed out state makes it nearly impossible to achieve total wellness—it simply does not work from a physiological standpoint. It is during the times of "rest and digest", when we are not under threat (no tigers, no jammed copy machines), that our bodies can truly heal.

Mediation and mindfulness allows us to drop down into that healing space, no matter where we are. What a wonderful thing! If you have never done any kind of meditation before, or never made time for quiet, uninterrupted reflection, it's time to look into a guided program to help get you started. There are dozens out there, most of them free, which can gently and slowly introduce you to the practice of meditation, podcasts, apps for phones and tablets, online classes and programs, and mp3 albums are all available to you. The general consensus says that you only need to do 10 minutes per day of these exercises to start seeing a benefit, and when you're faced with the choice of that, or hours spent in doctor's offices and pharmacies, let's just say it's no wonder that millions of people are establishing their own meditation routines every day.

It's okay if you're skeptical, but just be open to trying. Often the healing that happens from mindfulness is a very deep and subtle one, but it bolsters and enhances every other thing you do to help yourself. Yes, one session of meditation can bring some immediate relief, but just know that it will be short-lived. If you make it a regular routine, however, you will start to notice longer and more profound periods of peace and relaxation. You will start to sleep better, and may even find your insomnia becoming a thing of the past, especially if you practice right before bed or follow a special guided sleep meditation. You will notice that you are not as reactive to things that normally would upset you, like lost car keys or an overcrowded grocery store. You will find your interactions with other people are kinder and more productive, as you become less "on edge" and broaden your patience. You may also find that other healthy behaviors come more naturally to you, whether that's eating more vegetables, watching less television, or taking your dog on more walks. Your mind is the epicenter of all that you are and all you experience, so when you make improvements there, it's only natural to see a ripple effect into the rest of your life.

CHAPTER 9: GET YOUR EXERCISE ON!

Exercise is good in a variety of ways, so adding exercise to your schedule is very rarely a detriment in any way. It is a good idea to keep this in mind for all endeavors, as exercise helps with endorphins and better moods as well as weight loss efforts and improving your fight against obesity. Think of exercise as one part of your healthier lifestyle and regime, with diet as another critical aspect.

There's simply no excuse, in this day and age, for not getting enough exercise. Your doctor has probably told you to do it. Your gym teacher has definitely told you to do it. Maybe even your spouse or friend has made the not-so-gentle suggestion that you do it.

It's exercise, the thing that makes some people groan and pop out the leg rest on their couches, some people go out and buy expensive running shoes that they'll never use, and some people sign up for gym memberships. In our modern world, people react to the idea of exercise very differently, but generally it's because we have created such a level of pressure and expectation around it that it becomes overwhelming, so it seems easier to give up or just never try at all, but I will let you in on a little secret—you do not have to do exercise in order to get healthy – but it will certainly add to your armory.

Our society seems to have some pretty rigid rules when it comes to exercise, and there are plenty of people who will vehemently defend or deny that some forms of physical movement even count. Throw that nonsense away right now; you do not need to become a runner, a cyclist, a bodybuilder, a yoga nut or force yourself into any other athletic box. You can heal your body without any of those expectations and rules. You only need to give yourself permission to move your body in the way that feels good to you, and with enough regularity, your body will become stronger and healthier.

The instinct to move is one that is deeply embedded in us. Our ancestors walked for miles every day, they built shelters, hunted for food, and played with their loved ones. They did not have fancy treadmills or weight sets, personal trainers or triathlons. They just moved in the way that was natural for them, and so should you, and it does not have to be extremely strenuous or time consuming, in fact, this so-called "chronic cardio" is actually harmful to your health! You need to find a good balance where the amount of exercise is manageable for your lifestyle, but is also challenging enough to your system that it elicits change on a cellular level.

That's right—exercise is not just about burning calories or flattening your stomach. When you deliberately move your body, you are causing a powerful cascade of hormones and neurotransmitters through your brain and bloodstream, and over time, these physiological signals have the power to reverse diabetes, fight obesity, halt the progression of autoimmune diseases (and even reverse them!), and otherwise improve your quality of life. Yes, you may lose some weight and especially fat mass, and that's wonderful if that is one of your health goals, but don't get hung up on that being the only desirable outcome. Physical activity should be a means to show your body how much you appreciate it and want to help it along, not as a means of punishment. Sadly, many people in our society view it in this way, but you don't have to.

Nearly anything that gets your heart rate up and face flushed can be effective in your quest for health. Gardening, walking, yoga, tai chi, swimming—they're all wonderful ways to connect with your body and change yourself from the inside out, so if one of those speaks to you, then go for it! Or, if you are into group sports and love a pickup game of basketball or soccer, try to recruit some friends or coworkers for more regular meets, and if more hard-core individual pursuits are your thing, then run, ride, hike, and cross fit your way to a healthier body, just be sure to pay attention for symptoms of over-training. Heck, even popping in your headphones and dancing around the living room can be a wonderful way to release stress and get your blood pumping.

Depending on what your condition allows, try to aim for 4-5 exercise sessions per week. This seems to be the magic number where people experience the greatest benefits over time, without reaching burnout or exacerbating their symptoms. You can start small if you need to, those who have been sedentary for a long time and those suffering from chronic illnesses will need to implement a graded exercise routine until they are strong and fit enough for longer sessions, and mix things up if you get bored! Sign up for a new class at the rec center, try rock climbing, talk a friend into becoming a dance partner, or register for a local event. Whatever keeps you motivated and interested is what you should be doing, and it's okay if this changes periodically. Our bodies are incredible at adapting over time, so keep things fresh in order to take advantage of the greatest spectrum of healing power.

Now it may be that the idea of a weekly workout may be something that is not in your current routine. There is no need to think that the expectation on you is likely to be for you to leap straight into a daily hard pushing exercise regime – indeed, if you have not exercised for a while then this could be dangerous, and it is a good idea to visit a physician, health or exercise professional to ensure you do not overdo things early on. Having said that, it can be easy to make small changes to your regime – could you walk to the store down the block rather than jump in the car? Could you squeeze in walk around the block at lunchtime, or even a few lengths of a swimming pool? The chances are, once you build in exercise to your routine, you'll begin to want to protect that time – and will appreciate the many side benefits that regular exercise can bring. As we have discussed, it might also be the case that you can persuade a friend or colleague to join in with this part of your new routine – perhaps you'll find hat friends or colleagues have been thinking of starting to do something regular too – ask around – you might be pleasantly surprised!

As with diet it is important that any changes you make to your exercise regime are sustainable. This means that if you can find an activity you enjoy, but which is still giving you the benefits of exercise, then you are onto a winner. Exercise is good for the body and mind – if you can find a team sport, at a level appropriate to you, then you may find that the team ethos is something else you find you can enjoy.

Whilst we must stress that this is the sort of thing that you should run by your doctor, a sample workout plan could include:

Monday: 10 minutes of stretching followed by 60 minutes of walking or light jogging, followed by 10 further minutes of stretching.

Tuesday: 30 minute bike ride at a steady pace (ideal if around 14 miles per hour), followed by a 60 minute yoga class – this should be a faster paced yoga experience – we give more information on this later.

Wednesday: If you are feeling the push, take today to rest OR take a 20 minute walk at a pace of 20 minutes for each mile.

Thursday: 60 minutes of cycling indoors or outdoors, or 45 minutes of swimming, followed by 20 minutes of weight lifting. Note: if you cycled, focus on the arms, shoulders and abs while if you swam, you should focus the lifting on the legs and buttocks and core.

Friday: 20 minute run at 10 minutes per mile, followed by 60 minutes of yoga – again, this should be faster paced.

Saturday: 60 minutes of Zumba or a hike, followed by 20 minutes of workout, focused on the arms and shoulders and 10 minutes of stretching.

Sunday: Take today to rest OR take a 20 minute walk at a rate of 20 minutes per mile.

The other thing to bear in mind is how you track progress. It is unlikely you will be able to build such a routine straight into a normal functioning week for yourself, but if you can build in elements of it, more and more each week, then you will it easier to build your week around your exercise, rather than the other way around – as you get into your activity you are likely to want to do more and more of it anyway – exercise can be addictive like that! If you are able to keep a log of what you do, you can also look back to see what sense of achievement you can have related to what you have achieved. Recording your progress may seem embarrassing or discouraging at the beginning of your journey, but you will want those beginning weights, measurements, and pictures later to show yourself and others how far you have progressed. You might want to think about starting a blog either publicly or privately – this really can be a wonderful method to keeping track of your progress. Alternatively, you might want to keep a journal either on your computer or on paper as another great way to keep track. If you have a smartphone or tablet, you will find that there are any number of applications out there that can help you to keep track – some of them even calculate how far you have gone on exercise regimes and so on – use the technology! Once you begin to reach your goals and notice positive changes in your body, you are going to want to be able to compare your new self to your previous self. Always record your progress, no matter how small it may seem. This can help keep you on track to achieving your goals and help motivate you along the way.

The other thing to bear in mind with exercise is that it need not be a lonely occupation. Many people find that company can help with certain forms of exercise, or that the teamwork element of other sports can encourage people back again and again, as well as building in a social dimension – try and figure out what is likely to work best for you. Maybe you have exercised in the past but have let it go for whatever reason – try to think of the types of exercise you used to undertake that really got your juices flowing – and then see if you can recapture some of that – the chances are that you'll take to things you have done before more easily than trying to learn something completely new – of course the limits to what you might be able to do will have changed – and it is a good idea to consult a doctor before setting out on an exercise regime – but more than likely the things which you remember about being good about your chosen exercise will still be there, and you will likely find the memories flooding back too. There is really nothing to lose, so give it some thought, and get out there (or in there – you can do plenty at home)!

Tip : A Simple Exercise Program

Getting some exercise will not only make you healthier, you'll find that your energy levels are higher, your mood is improved, and you'll just generally feel better!

We have already explored that it might be difficult to think about how you can build exercise into your life. If that is how you are feeling, then here are some easy to follow exercise plans, to help you get there!

With any workout, make sure that you take 2–5 minutes to stretch, limber up and get a little warm. Run in place, do some pushups, and just make sure that you're ready to take on a little bit of exercise. This does not have to be extensive, just a warm-up to wake up your body.

You will need a jump rope. These are not expensive, and you can find them at your local big-box retailer, online, or just about anywhere. Find a good jump rope, and you will be ready to take on this 20 minute cardio plan.

Do not skip the jump rope.

It is going to be your major tool in this option. It can be as low as 99 cents in some places. You don't need the best one in the world, you just need one to start.

Chin-up Bar/Pull-up Bar

You'll also need to purchase a chin-up bar or similar contraption for your doorframe. Otherwise, go to a park or gym that has ine that you can use; most major parks in metropolitan areas will have one. If you can't find one, look for monkey bars or a jungle gym that you can use, instead. Chin-up bars and equipment that fit in a door frame can cost anywhere from $5 - $30 and can help you with a variety of exercises. If you can't find one, look for a pull-up bar option that also can be placed in the frame of a doorway. These too are cost effective.

20 Minute Cardio Cycles

This routine should be done no less than 3 days a week. Later, it can be combined with weight training or resistance training routines mentioned before or after this section. Don't do this daily, and make sure to rest if you're working out 6 days a week.

24 Squats

To do a squat, plant your feet firmly on the ground no more than shoulder distance apart. Bend your knees without bending your back, keeping a sense of straightness to the back and then lower yourself into a squat and rise back up again to a standing position. 24 squats will get you started.

40 Chin-ups or 40 Pull-ups

Do 40 chin-ups, or as many as you can to start. On day 1 you may not be able to get this done swiftly, so don't worry. Do as many as you can to get you started.

For those who don't have a chin-up bar, pull-ups will also work. Your goal is 40 total.

Jump Rope

After you've done the routine described above, or have hit around the 10 minute mark, you will want to jump rope. Jump for the rest of your time, no matter how much time you have left. 40 chin-ups or pull-ups should not take you 20 minutes, or even close to it. However, if it does get close, stop what you're doing, get to your jump rope and finish the workout that way.

Things to Remember About This Workout

The goal of this work out is to have at least 10 minutes dedicated to the first couple of steps, and 10 minutes dedicated to jumping rope. You can mix and match how you want to do this, as some may want to start with jumping rope.

You may find it silly at first, but jumping rope for 10 minutes straight through may be one of the hardest cardiovascular exercises that you'll try. The combination of muscle and resistance training here will be a nice beginning to build on.

For Experts (mix things up)

When you feel that this workout is not getting you as pumped as it once did, change your days and start a new routine with weight training. Every other day should be dedicated to lifting weights and light cardiovascular exercises, while this routine should be performed on alternate days. The overall goal is to have you work out 6 days a week and rest one full day. Combined with a good nutritional diet, and even supplements, this is a total body workout that will give you some serious results.

Do not forget to rest at least one day. Resting allows for muscle recovery.

Quick Tips

You're not going to master these routines in a single day. Each one may seem easy, but if you follow the correct forms and cycle through 40 reps of each and then jump rope or vice-versa, you will find it tiring. If it's too easy, double up your reps, and try to allow for 10 minutes of constant rope jumping. Just 10 minutes of jumping rope will help you get the results you want in terms of weight loss, but the added elements will give you a bit of muscle training to mix things up.

Keep a few extra things in mind:

Do not try to do it all on day 1. Routines like this take time to master.

Do not forget the jump rope and chin-up/pull-up bar.

Do not give up if you can't fit it all in. Try your best.

Do try different variations on this.

Do add weight to your squats over time.

Do share your knowledge and results with friends and family.

Now it may be that your limits have changed substantially from when you used to exercise – there is something for everyone however, and it may be that you want to consider something more gentle – and some would say holistic, that is it affects a few parts of your body and helps them work together – and that something is yoga. This needn't see you having to don special kit or even needing a special mat or anything – many yoga moves can be learned and undertaken in the privacy of your own home. Yoga is a hobby that helps lower stress levels and improve bodily processes simply by refocusing energy and distracting your mind from the various issues it goes over repeatedly on a daily basis.

One great way to work meditation and yoga into your daily life is to plan on a period of time where you can complete the following exercises and then segue right into your seated meditation session, thereby calming yourself and extending that period where you are focusing on physical sensations and being in the moment, rather than being lost in a mental list of stresses and worries. Again though, much better to introduce some of these elements to your everyday, and try to increase them as you go along rather than concede defeat as you don't have time to follow every aspect through. There are lots and lots of great resources available on yoga, both online and in books – have an explore at your local library or on yoga websites to see what might suit you and your circumstances.

For many people, yoga can become a way of life – something that transcends many other aspects of their lives – it can help them think more clearly, feel more supple, and help to strengthen their core areas – you might find you are hooked if you try it – that would be no bad thing .Bear in mind though, that you don't need to go to a formal class – you can try out many of the simpler moves in the confines of your own home.

As with other elements we have discussed, relating to exercise and diet, it may be that you do not have time to work in the type of structured approach we have suggested above. In that case, the same principle applies- it is better to try and get started on some of these elements than just say you don't have time and throw the baby out with the bathwater. See, for example, if you are able to draw in some of the elements of meditation to your everyday existence – that might be the option of factoring in some aspect of this to your everyday routine, maybe by focusing on your breathing rhythms whilst on public transport as part of your daily commute, or escaping to a private meeting room for ten minutes in the middle of a cluttered and busy day – take some time out for yourself and see if it makes a difference.

CONCLUSION

If you are able to take one thing away from this book, it is that there is always an element of control that you can take – if you feel that the symptoms you are showing relate to Leaky Gut Syndrome then, as we have made clear, proponents assert that there is a lot that you can do yourself to try and make for a more robust underlying system – which in turn can lead to a healthier digestive system. In this book we have explored what Leaky Gut Syndrome is considered to be, the opinions of medical and other practitioners, but also sought to give you some ideas as to what you can do yourself to improve your digestive and wider health. Of course many of these ideas are not necessarily new – thinking about diet, exercise, mental wellbeing – but by picking up this book and trying to learn more about Leaky Gut Syndrome and how it might be affecting your life, then it may be that you are able to take one, two or all of these tracks to see if making changes can improve how you feel overall.

SO then, we have explored what proponents of Leaky Gut Syndrome say that the condition is, and how it manifests itself – that is what the symptoms are. It is considered that Leaky Gut Syndrome, described as an intestinal permeability ailment, can cause many health problems, psychological and physical. While many of the symptoms can be vague, we have explored how taking control of how you monitor your own body and the symptoms which you are experiencing – and how you note these down – can help when you have discussions with your doctor or others you choose to help you. Not only can such an approach help these practitioners, it can also ensure you have an accurate log of how things have changed over time – of course you may want to link monitoring of your symptoms with your diet and also your exercise regime – they are all linked in some way, and you may be able to identify some useful patterns.

We have also explored the scenario that because some of the symptoms associated with digestive issues can be vague, and it is not always apparent how they might link with each other, then so it could be the case that doctors or other qualified medical practitioners may have trouble diagnosing and prescribing the correct treatment for your particular condition, it may seem apparent to you that you have what proponents describe as Leaky Gut Syndrome, but in order to give your doctor the best chance to help you, then it is best to collate as much relevant information as you possibly can. Furthermore, however, much of the advice in this book can be useful for all sorts of other reasons, and the ideas it contains are considered to be useful for anyone to follow, even if you don't have Leaky Gut Syndrome.

Through a better and healthier diet which consists of mainly fruits and vegetables, you can begin to improve digestive issues. Detoxing is a great way for anyone to rid themselves of harmful toxins and bacteria that have passed into the blood stream through overly permeable intestinal walls. After completing your two week detox, you should begin to feel great and lose many symptoms including bloat, diarrhea, constipation, and even headaches. It is to be hoped that the recipe suggestions and meal plan hit the mark for you, but remember that herbs are always a healthy and tasty addition to most recipes.

While Leaky Gut Syndrome is not considered a medical term – in that it is not recognised by many health professionals, it is nonetheless certainly considered an important issue by others, and one that requires more investigation. It is important therefore to regulate your diet if experiencing the symptoms of Leaky Gut Syndrome – we have explored this in some detail, but it is worth a reminder that decisions you take around your diet can be good for your physical and mental wellbeing – all of this contributes to you having a more robust system, and that is something to which we should all aspire. In addition to eating healthily, we have also considered some of the supplemental ways that some proponents believe can help to treat and ease the symptoms of Leaky Gut

Syndrome. Again, many of these interventions can be good for you for wider reasons – but it is important to reiterate, that if you are suffering from the types of symptoms we describe in the book, then you should seek the opinion of a qualified doctor in the first instance.

This stands to reason. Of course, it's always a good idea to follow the advice of a health care professional when taking new steps with your health. However we have made the point that you can take control yourself – not least by monitoring and logging what is going on with your symptoms, diet and exercise, and cross referencing those to changes in how you feel overall. If you can identify some trends yourself then it makes things that much easier for those from whom you choose to seek help, advice or medication. By working with your doctor, therapist, and following the advice in this book, you will begin to see results concerning your Leaky Gut Syndrome symptoms.

In this book, we have also taken a look at more ways you can improve your general health, and given you some tips on how to make this more than a cleanse, and turn it into a complete lifestyle change. If you will follow the advice in this book, then it's highly likely that your health will improve in many ways, not just in the elimination of Leaky Gut Syndrome. We hope that by putting this information into practice in your daily life, you will be able to enjoy living long and with good health for all of your days.

All of the issues we have covered might be relevant to your situation – but the most important thing to take on board is that you can take control. Hopefully this book will have triggered some useful ideas, or been the prompt for you to speak to someone about your particular issues. One thing to bear in mind is that you are not alone in being in a position where you are suffering from the types of symptoms we have described in this book. Nor are you the first to try and find out more about what may be underlying these conditions, and , of course, what you might be able to do about it. This means the route has been well trodden – and who knows, if you start to talk about your thoughts, wishes and so on with those around you then you are likely to find support, but more than that, you might find that others close to you have experienced, or are even experiencing, something similar. This is one of those areas that people can feel they don't really want to talk about with others, but it might very well be that that is absolutely the best thing that you can choose to do.

So, there are options open to you – you can choose to go and see qualified individuals, you can learn to monitor your own situation more accurately, you can take control of your diet and exercise regime – but most of all you can choose to take more control of your situation. It is to be hoped that reading this book helps you along the road on that journey. Good luck!

Made in the USA
San Bernardino, CA
09 October 2018